Gym Hater's Guide to Fitness

By J. M. Burnett

ISBN: 1500979929
ISBN-13: 978-1500979928

Dedication

This book is dedicated to all of us who
would like to be healthier, but have no desire to
join the ranks of the "gym rats.

Contents

I don't really hate gyms; they just aren't for me

I suppose I should set one thing straight before we begin. I don't hate gyms. I've actually belonged to a few, gone a few times, then stopped. I once even attended a women's only gym for about 10 months, three times a week. I saw results, but the minute my schedule changed and it became inconvenient, I just never managed to get back.

It's true that I'm not a "gym rat" and never will be. I don't like to exercise…or sweat…or wear fitness attire in public.

What's also true, though, is that I know I need more

exercise in order to be healthy. The irony, for me, is that I've worked in the health and wellness sector for almost a decade now…and I get exceedingly tired of hearing how getting healthy, or even getting fit, equates to going to the gym.

It doesn't.

We're going to talk more about how fitness and gyms don't necessarily go together, but first I want to vent a little about the fitness industry as well as the blinders that have been securely fastened on so many of us by the fitness industry, the fashion industry, the media, and the unending social pressure to be thin and perpetually young.

First, thin doesn't necessarily equal healthy.

Far too many young girls develop eating disorders by trying to emulate fashion models and celebrities. Many of those in the fashion industry have come clean about the unhealthy lifestyles of models who live on coffee and diet soda, smoke, and rarely eat a healthy diet in order to stay thin. Sure, there are exceptions, but the reality is that most of us cannot either achieve or maintain a size zero and still be healthy. It's way past time that we accept that the human body comes in a variety of shapes and sizes, and that's a good thing.

Second, the fitness industry is just that – an industry, and like any industry they exist to sell you something.

We're going to talk about the dollars and cents of that industry (briefly) in just a second, but let's all agree first that good health and even fitness can be achieved without perfect abs or the ability to survive the latest boot camp class. When we talk about fitness, we're talking about health...not image.

So what is the fitness industry selling? The messaging and advertising would make you think it's all about perfect abs and toned bodies and, let's face it...sex sells. What the fitness industry is really selling is quite different.

They're selling memberships.

And, even more importantly, they're selling most people memberships that they pay for *and almost never use.*

According to 2014 statistics published by fitness industry authority IHRSA (International Health, Racquet & Sportsclub Association), almost 16% of Americans own a fitness center membership. Of those, *67% are unused.* In fact, the industry depends on those members who pay, but don't show up. Few clubs have the square footage and equipment to actually serve all of their members. They know that they may be crowded in January, when everyone makes that fresh New Years' resolution, but that it will begin to empty out and get back to normal about February.

Think about that for a second.

That means about 58 million people have fitness center memberships, and almost 39 million of those don't use them.

Since the average U.S. fitness center membership, according to IHRSA, is $58 – higher in urban areas and at upscale clubs, and lower in rural areas – that means we are essentially flushing away more than **$2 billion** each and every year.

An individual paying $58 a month for a membership they don't use is wasting $696 a year. That will buy you a modest, but relaxing weekend get-away, or a car payment or two. In my household, that would be groceries for about a month and a half.

So why don't people just cancel their memberships?

Guilt? That feeling that "I should go"? The finality that cancelling the membership almost feels like they're giving up on the whole idea of getting fit?

I'm sure the reasons are different from person to person, but the industry counts on those feelings…the ones that keep you paying good money for nothing.

Here's something else to consider. Remember that 16% figure? If 16% of Americans have fitness center memberships, then 84% of us do not.

Clearly, gyms just aren't for everyone.

In fact, we're in the majority.

Does that mean that we don't care about getting fit and healthy? Absolutely not.

For many people, the cost of a membership is prohibitive. For others, their days are already overburdened with responsibilities and time is too tight to allow for a trip to the gym.

In fact, of those gym members who actually go, the average number of visits a week is just two.

Clearly, it's hard for all of us to get to the gym.

The irony & the Amish

As I said, I've worked in the health and wellness field for almost a decade now. As part of that work, I often had to visit fitness centers.

Now, I know that my sense of the ironic is highly tuned, but it never ceased to make me laugh when I'd see people at the gym circling the parking lot to find the closest possible parking spot...in order to go inside and get on the treadmill.

How about those who would take the elevator up in order to get on the stair climber?

Or what about the members that complained at the front desk that their exercise class had been moved to the studio "all the way at the far end of the building"?

It would be funny if it was once or twice, but these were normal occurrences!

Part of the reason we are growing less healthy as a culture, that chronic illnesses like diabetes and heart disease are increasing, is that we have virtually all severed ourselves from actual physical work. We sit in our cars to go places. We sit at our desks and at our computers at work. And when we return home, mentally stressed from our day but having had no physical outlet, we sit on our couches in front of our television sets to relax.

Please note that I'm saying "we" here. I'm not pointing fingers. I'm in the same boat.

Sure, there are some of us who have physically demanding jobs, but those numbers are dwindling as more and more of us work with our minds instead of our bodies.

In contrast, I was fascinated to read about a pedometer study (conducted in 2004 by Dr. Bassett) conducted among the Old Order Amish. Since the Amish do not use electricity or modern devices (like cars, tractors, dishwashers and vacuum cleaners), they do a lot more physical activity in the course of their day than the non-Amish population. In fact, the study showed that the average Amish woman walked the equivalent of 14,196 steps a day, and the average Amish man did 18,425 steps a day.

Now, I'm not going to trade in my car for a horse anytime soon, nor am I going to call the utility company to pull the plug on my electrical service. I'm not suggesting you should either…so don't panic!

What's particularly interesting is that, despite a diet that is fairly high in baked goods and fried foods (and averages 4,000 calories a day), the Amish have low rates of heart disease and diabetes – two of the biggest killers in modern America.

When the Amish do develop heart disease or diabetes, it is generally much later in life – when advancing age results in a more sedentary lifestyle. Until then, the high level of activity the Amish engage in daily garners them significant health benefits.

There are also much lower rates of overweight and obesity among Old Order Amish who live in this traditional way. In fact, Dr. Bassett's study (of adults aged 18 to 75) showed overweight in only about ¼ of the population and obesity in 0% of the men, and only 9% of women.

By contrast, more than 34% of American adults age 20 and over are overweight, and 35% are obese (according to the Centers for Disease Control).

By now, we've probably all heard the recommendation that walking 10,000 steps a day helps us to achieve better health. That seems to be in line with the Amish pedometer study's findings, and is probably a good guideline. In fact, there's another whole new segment of the fitness industry growing up to provide you with wearable, digital activity monitors and flashy websites to help you track those steps and encourage you to take more.

I'm not slamming the devices and the websites, but I question how necessary they are. You don't see the Amish wearing them, do you?

In our culture, there is tremendous pressure to buy….to buy everything, including fitness center memberships and the latest wearable devices. But, like many of the things we are persuaded to buy, they aren't really necessary at all. You can achieve better health and fitness very simply. And, no, I'm not advising you to adopt an Amish lifestyle, to set up a home gym, or even to start an exercise routine at home.

I'm not even suggesting that you go for a daily one hour walk.

In fact, in a time when money is tight for many of us, and the concept of "free time" sounds like a not very funny joke, what I'm suggesting will enhance your health, improve your fitness, save you money, and even make you feel an enhanced sense of peace in your own home.

I promise.

Let's talk about steps

The 10,000 steps a day recommendation is a good one, but is it really a "one size fits all" solution? It's been shown to make a difference in overall health, and even to aid in weight loss. For those who haven't heard about it before, 10,000 steps a day equals approximately 5 miles for the average person. If you were to set out to walk 5 miles, it would take most of us 2 to 2-1/2 hours. I don't know about your schedule, but that doesn't fit in mine.

There's some good news, though. The average person

already travels anywhere from 2,000 to 5,000 steps in their daily routine. Numbers vary tremendously depending on which studies you look at, as well as where in the country (or world) you live. Overall, Americans tend to walk less than other countries, and residents of suburban areas walk less than city dwellers.

For those of us who would like to lose some weight, it's also good to know that obese people tend to walk less than those of normal weight. Which is cause and which is effect is less clear.

But I said I wasn't going to tell you to go for a walk every day, right? Right.

I'm not saying "don't go for a walk" – because going for a walk is a wonderful thing. It gets you outside, moving, and in the fresh air. That's a good thing. There's also something very meditative about walking that can help our mood, as well as giving us uninterrupted time to think…something that rarely happens in our average day.

What I do know, though, is that finding the time to go walk for an hour, or even a half hour, can be challenging with everything else we have to do.

But first, back to steps and the idea of activity levels. The recommendation for 10,000 steps a day grew out of a number of studies and public health discussions. One of the important studies, however, was that same 2004 Amish pedometer study conducted by Dr. Bassett.

Dr. Bassett did not recommend any particular number of steps for good health. Rather, he broke down daily activity levels as follows:

- Less than 2,500 steps = basal activity (basically the incidental movement that most people do to survive...make and eat food, shower, get dressed, etc.
- 2,500 to 4,999 steps = limited activity
- 5,000 to 7,499 steps = low activity
- 7,500 to 9,999 steps = somewhat active
- 10,000 to 12,499 steps = active
- More than 12,500 steps = highly active

More importantly, follow up studies to Dr. Bassett's original findings showed that the greatest health benefits were gained simply by moving up even just one activity level.

In other words, 10,000 steps isn't necessarily the "one size fits all" solution that we're being told it is. It's just enough to get us to the bottom of the "active" rating.

The other recommendation currently being circulated is that everyone should be getting 150 minutes a week of moderate level exercise or 75 minutes a week of vigorous exercise. Naturally, this is a good thing for our health and our weight. It also implies that we need to work out at a gym, or go running, or take up some other vigorous activity like martial arts or boxing. This simply isn't true either.

What I'm suggesting, and following myself, is a plan to get the movement we need, to meet the moderate or vigorous activity level recommended, and not waste precious money and time doing it.

The most important fitness equipment you probably already own

For our purposes, there's only one piece of fitness equipment you need to own, and you probably already do.

I'm not talking about a treadmill or a home gym, or even a pedometer (although one of those can be handy if you're interested in tracking your progress).

I'm actually talking about a timer...like the kind you probably already have on your kitchen stove or your cellphone.

What will you be timing? Exercise sessions? Nope.

Think back to that Amish study. The Amish aren't doing aerobics or weight lifting. They're doing the tasks that need to be done to make their lives happen.

And that's what I want you to do.

No, you aren't going to be plowing fields or shoveling out the pig pen. You will be doing more of what you need to do to keep yourself healthy and your daily life working smoothly.

Let me tell you a little more about how I came to this place in my personal "fitness journey." For most of the last 18 years, I've been a single mother, working, sometimes going to school, sometimes managing rental properties. I had no time for a gym, and no energy to take up a regular exercise program. There was also the issue of self-discipline…something that I would need in spades in order to keep up an exercise program on my own.

In fact, most weeks, I worked hard and dealt with a great deal of stress, but most of my work was done at a computer or in meetings, and not with my body.

By the time I got home, made dinner, oversaw homework, and spent some time with my son…I was exhausted. The evening hours saw me in front of the TV, or with a book, or writing (another passion), all of which kept me sitting and barely moving.

Meanwhile, housework got pushed to the weekend (and I spent a lot of time wishing I could afford to hire someone to do it for me); yard work got put off longer and longer and only done when it was an absolutely necessity. The car got taken to the car wash.

You see where I'm going here, right?

The reality is that movement is movement – whether we're doing it in a fitness class at the gym or mowing the lawn. I knew that, of course, I just never thought about it much.

But here's what's true: The activities that we do to make our houses clean and our yards beautiful, to grow some of our own food in a garden, these all add up to the exercise that builds fitness and good health.

In fact, here are some examples:

- Grocery shopping = 67 steps per minute (that's 4,020 an hour)
- Light housework = 72 steps per minute (4,320 an hour)
- Vacuuming = 101 steps per minute (6,060 an hour)
- Sweeping and mopping floors = 51 steps per minute (3060 an hour)

And, outside, the same holds true:

- Washing the car = 87 steps per minute (5,220 per hour)
- Gardening = 116 steps per minute (6,960 per hour)
- Mowing (with a push mower, not a ride on!) = 160 steps a minute (9,600 an hour)
- Raking leaves = 125 steps per minute (7,500 an hour)
- General yard work = 145 steps per minute (8,700 per hour)

One of the primary reasons we are so unhealthy in America is that we don't move enough. And yet, many of us hire others to do these activities for us…spending money that we could better use elsewhere or put into our savings account, while we get less and less healthy for lack of movement.

We know it's true, don't we?

It's a paradox of modern life in America that we are unhealthy for lack of movement, pay others to do these kinds of activities for us, and then pay to join a fitness center (which most of us don't use) to get the exercise we know we need.

Here's my suggestion: Cut that nonsense out!

I made a commitment to get the steps I need, as well as meet the guidelines for vigorous/moderate exercise, without spending money to do it. As a result, I am healthier, my house is cleaner, and my yard is tidier…and I'm saving money as well.

What I needed was a plan. The beauty of this plan is that it has the side benefit of immediate gratification. You house looks and feels better. Your yard is beautiful and welcoming. Maybe you even get some fresh, homegrown produce to serve to your family.

So, what's the plan?

Here's the plan...first steps

Our goal is to move up our activity level – one step at a time.

If you have a pedometer and you want to track your normal level for a week to see where your actual starting point is, please go right ahead.

If you don't have a pedometer and want to do this, by all means, go ahead. Just keep in mind that there's no need to spend $50 to $100 on a fancy digital model that connects to an online program. A simple pedometer, available for a few dollars, is more than enough.

If you don't have a pedometer and just want to get started...fantastic! Let's go!

You'll need to decide what activities work for you.

Condo or apartment dwellers may not have a yard to work in, so those activities might be out for you. I'm going to assume that most of us work a full-time job, during the day, but please customize to fit your own schedule.

When you get home tomorrow, I want you to set your stove or phone timer for 30 minutes. Immediately start cleaning. It can be sweeping and mopping, dusting, washing windows, cleaning the bathroom – whatever needs it most. You can stay in one room or move all over the house. But you will keep moving for 30 minutes, and clean until the timer goes off. Once it does, you're done. Your house will be a little cleaner, and all that you've lost is the 30 minutes that you normally spend collapsed on the couch or mulling over what needs to be done.

If you have kids, tell them they can make a choice. They can do homework until the timer goes off, or they can clean too. Movement is good for kids as well – and so is learning to take some responsibility for the home they live in. Most of us don't work alongside our kids very often, and it's a good life lesson for them.

It's that simple.

In 30 minutes, depending on what activity you choose, you'll get in anywhere from 1,500 to 3,000 steps. Since Dr. Bassett's activity levels are done in 2,500 step intervals, just 30 minutes of housework a day may be enough to move you up a level.

Do this every day. Inside or outside doesn't matter. On days when you're putting in your 30 minutes outside, you'll probably be getting a few more steps in – averaging 2,500 to 4,000. **The key is to keep moving. Do not stop.**

The first step is truly that simple.

For most of us, that won't be enough, but start there with 30 minutes of steady housework or yard work a day in addition to what you normally do right now.

Second steps...

Some of you may want to take a little more aggressive steps, or find that 30 minutes a day surprisingly easy to achieve. If that's you, you can set the timer for 45 minutes, or perhaps add in an additional session of 15 or 30 minutes at another point of the day.

Ideally, we'll all get to an additional hour of activity a day – bringing us up two levels from where we were when we started.

What about that other fitness criteria?

Remember that other fitness criteria? The one that says we all need 150 minutes a week of moderate intensity exercise or 75 minutes of vigorous exercise?

Once you've gotten comfortable with the 30 minutes a day, work on stepping up the intensity. Move faster at whatever you're doing. Moderate intensity means that you could talk as you do your activity, but not sing.

To get to vigorous intensity, add in some tougher activities – dig up a garden or landscape borders, scrub a floor vigorously with a scrub brush, do something requiring more lifting and bending and do it at a good pace. Add in some weight lifting…if you're cleaning out the kitchen cabinets, add in some bicep curls and tricep extensions with your canned goods as you put them away again. Squat down to scrub the baseboards, stand up to move to the next section and squat down again to scrub.

Alternatively, keep up your normal 30 minutes of activity, cleaning in the house or working in the yard. Pick your slowest day of the week, and add in a 25 minutes session of vigorous activity on that weekday and on both Saturday and Sunday.

If you have space, putting in a garden is a wonderful way to get in some vigorous exercise – digging, hoeing and weeding. It has the side benefit of producing some healthy vegetables for you and your family, and providing a healthy dose of fresh air and sunlight as well.

Be a bad waitress

When I was working my way through college, I spend a lot of time waitressing. I was trained by a woman who had waitressed for years, and her primary message to new servers (other than take care of your customers and be nice to them), was to never waste a trip. We were all supposed to always have our hands full, so that we didn't waste a step.

That makes sense for servers, but for our purposes, it's bad advice. My advice to you: Be a Bad Waitress.

Oftentimes, we'll pile things up at the bottom of the stairs in order to take them all up at the same time later, or set things aside to take out to the car, into the garage, or even into another room so that we can make a single trip.

Instead, make lots of trips. If you have something in your hand that needs to go to another place – take it there right now. Don't worry about being efficient – in fact, efficiency in moving is what's killing us now. We need to move more, not less.

Add to this the advice we've all heard to take the stairs and not the elevator, to park as far as possible from the entrance to our destination, to get up and move on commercials when we're watching TV. These are all good things to increase our level of incidental exercise, and that can make a real difference to the number of steps we take in a day.

We all know that one person who "never sits still" right? Generally, those people don't have as much trouble maintaining a healthy weight as those of us who can sit for hours, and their base level of steps is higher than the average as well.

My son, who is 17, is a gaming fanatic. He can comfortably spend hours sitting at his computer – working on his schoolwork, and also playing games and Skyping with friends. He should be unfit, but he isn't. The reason for that is simple – he's a walker. When he's thinking, he walks laps around the outside perimeter of our swimming pool. When he's on the phone, he'll lap around the yard or walk around the house. Despite hours in front of the computer, his perpetual walking keeps him slim and fit.

You can accomplish the same thing, even if you aren't one of those "can't sit still" people. If you watch TV in the evening, get up at every commercial break and spend it de-cluttering. Simply grab the first thing you see that needs to be put away and take it to wherever it belongs. While you're at the first item's destination, grab the first thing you see there that's out of place and take it where it belongs. Repeat until your show is back on.

For those of us who don't watch TV (with commercials anyway), set your timer for 15 minutes after dinner to de-clutter and tidy. The additional steps will add to your total for the day.

For those who read instead of watching TV, set your timer at the end of every chapter. In fact, go set your timer for 15 minutes right now and have a little "bad waitress" session. No doubt there's something in the room you're in right now that needs to be put away.

Go do it.

But what about my kids?

As a single mom, one of the things that made it challenging to go to the gym, or even for a walk, was my son. Sure, when he was small enough to go in a stroller I could take him for a walk with me, but leaving him to go to the gym after I'd already left him all day to work just wasn't something I was comfortable with.

I'm not faulting those that do. There's a certain "put on your own oxygen mask first" quality about taking time for yourself and your own health and fitness. I still struggled though.

Our current reality in America though is that our

children are fat and getting fatter. Childhood obesity is a serious problem, and experts suggest that this generation of children will have more serious illnesses and shorter lifespans than their parents did. Type 2 diabetes (which used to be called "adult onset") is on the rise among young children and teenagers, as are elevated blood pressure and high cholesterol. Is this what we want for our children?

Your kids need to get up and move as much as you do.

My recommendation: Include your entire family in this exercise. When you set the timer, everyone cleans, or works in the yard...even if it's as simple as picking up and putting away toys and clothes, or raking leaves into a pile to jump in later. It is good for our children to learn what's involved in running a household, and to learn an appreciation for the things their parents do to keep that household running smoothly. At the same time, they're moving their bodies and learning new skills. Even very young children can sweep, empty wastebaskets and dust. They are particularly handy for washing baseboards, since they're already down there (and, no, I'm not kidding). If you use non-toxic cleaners like vinegar water, then you don't have to worry about their safety.

Make a weekend ritual to wash the car together...bucket of soapy water, sponges, hose and all. Yes, they'll make a mess and you'll all get wet. You'll also probably have a lot of fun (once you get past the initial disbelief and whining). Remember, washing the car nets you each 87 steps a minute. If you spend half an hour doing it, you've earned 2,610 steps – and moved yourselves up an activity level.

Here's the one time I'll tell you to go for a walk

Go take a walk, as a family. Grab the stroller, the dog, the kids…everyone goes. Don't get in the car, just go out your front door and walk. Explore your neighborhood together. Heck, maybe you'll even meet some of your neighbors.

Talk about their day. Talk about school. Let them hear about your day and your work. Check out the neighbors' yards and talk about what you might like to plant in your own.

So few of us actually have conversations with our children. We direct them through their day – do this, don't do that, do your homework, wash your hands, brush your teeth….but we don't talk about what they think. There's huge value in that.

As a plus, walking at a normal pace earns you 100 steps a minute. That half hour walk (after dinner is an ideal time), earns you each 3,000 steps, and moves you up another activity level.

Have fun as a family

Instead of watching TV together or going to a movie, do something physical with your family. Go bowling, crank up the tunes and dance in the living room, or go bicycling. Doing activities together is great for your family – and great for your fitness. Remember, getting the equivalent of 2,500 steps moves you up an activity level.

Here's a sampling:

- Dancing = 93 steps a minute (5,580 an hour)
- Line dancing (go ahead, teach them the Electric Slide) = 139 steps a minute (8,340 an hour)
- Bicycling at a leisurely pace = 100 steps a minute (6,000 an hour)
- Bowling = 87 steps a minute (more if you don't sit down but stand up and cheer for each other instead, 5,220 an hour)
- Golfing, without a cart = 122 steps a minute (7,329 an hour)

Set your goal to do something fun and physical together for an hour at least once each weekend. You'll all be better off for it.

The same applies with our friends. How many of us have friendships that revolve around getting together to sit, eat and drink? Instead, suggest some of the activities above, or at least a post-dinner stroll. Oftentimes it's simply habit that keeps us immobile. Start a new tradition instead.

How it all comes together

Does it seem too simple?

I know it did for me.

Just remember that it pays for everyone in the fitness industry to make it sound complicated. According to them, not only do you need a membership, but also a personal trainer and some special clothes and equipment, and probably some special protein drinks or whatever the latest fad is, too.

They make it sound that way because they're trying to

sell you something. The fitness industry is almost a $22 billion a year industry. In fact, IHRSA said that last year, fitness industry revenue was $21,800,000,000. That's a lot of zeroes. Clearly, they're selling a lot of people a lot of stuff.

The fitness magazines, women's magazines and health-promoting TV shows all need a new story every edition or every episode – so there's always something else to buy.

It's time for a reality check.

The Amish are healthier than the general public is – despite butter and bacon and cake. They are healthier because they move their bodies. They haven't mechanized or hired out the work of living. They do it, with their own bodies and their own hands.

I'm not saying we all need to go back to the land. But we do need to stop sitting on the couch.

So, how does this all look?

Here's the plan:

- Step 1: If you have a pedometer and/or care to, go ahead and measure your normal activity level every day for a week. Write it down somewhere, and then stop worrying about it. (Feel free to skip this step if you aren't a person who likes to keep track of everything). **– 0 steps**

- Step 2: Add in the 30 minute housework/yard work

session every day after work and on the weekend. Pick whatever activity you want, just keep moving until the timer goes off. **– Average 2,500 steps. Congratulations, you just moved up 1 activity level and garnered some health benefits!** (Your house is probably cleaner too, right?)

- Step 3: Aim for hitting the exercise intensity recommendations of 150 minutes a week of moderate intensity exercise by upping the speed and intensity of your housework so that talking is possible, but singing is not. Alternatively, you can select 3 days a week to do a 25 minute sessions of vigorous activity – shoveling, hoeing, "stand and squat" baseboard scrubbing. **– Congratulations, you just increased your fitness by adding more intensity to your workout!**

- Step 4: Add in a 15 minute "bad waitress" session every day. Just walk around and put things where they go. If you have no clutter, feel free to dust! - **Average 1,500 steps.** Hey, why not make it 25 minutes and move up another activity level?

- Step 5: Add in some family fun, or friends fun, on the weekend to up your activity level. Spend an hour going for a walk, or bowling, or dancing. You'll earn anywhere from 6,000 to 8,000 steps and really up your activity level. Feeling hardcore? Do an hour on Saturday **and** Sunday instead of just one.

Want to take it up a notch?

Once you've gotten accustomed to the basic steps, you may find yourself wanting to do more. If that's the case, consider:

- Make your housework/ yard work time an hour instead of 30 minutes. It takes a bigger commitment of time, but you'll also up your activity by an average of 5,000 steps a day – two activity levels!

- Add an after dinner walk (with family or by yourself). Half an hour of walking helps regulate blood sugar, boosts metabolism, and earns you 3,000 steps and one activity level.

- Put in a garden. If you have a yard, even a small garden will give you opportunities to hoe, dig, weed…earning you steps, lots of bending and stretching, and some fresh produce too.

- Have a physical weekend project. Take the opportunity to do a special project on weekends that doesn't involve sitting on the couch. Clean out and organize a closet, paint a wall or a room, do a deep clean on a room.

The couch is not your friend

Every study in modern America shows that we need to move more and sit less. The best exercise we can do is simply to get off the couch, and move our bodies. Sweep a room, walk around the block, wash the dog, mow the lawn, wash the car, or organize your junk drawer...anything that gets you on your feet instead of on your butt.

It's that simple.

Often, we are our own worst enemies by over

complicating things. We think that getting fit and healthy means going to a gym, having a personal trainer, taking some special supplements. In reality, the secrets to good health aren't secret at all. Get some fresh air and sunshine. Move. Drink water. Eat real food.

My wish for you is that you don't buy into the hype. Save your fitness center membership money for a vacation or your retirement, or to go bowling with your family.

Just move. If you want to be healthy, then the couch is not your friend.